Taking Control OF Hypertension

A Comprehensive Guide to Lowering Your Blood Pressure

Dr. Thomas K. McGlynn

Copyright © 2023 Dr. Thomas K. McGlynn

All rights reserved. No part of this book may be reproduced, stored in a retrieval system, or transmitted in any form or by any means, electronic, mechanical, photocopying, recording, or otherwise, without the prior written permission of the copyright owner.

This book is intended for informational purposes only and please consult with a healthcare professional for personalized medical advice.

The author has made every effort to ensure the accuracy of the information contained in this book as of the date of publication. However, the information contained in this book is subject to change without notice and the author make no commitment to update the information contained in this book.

TABLE OF CONTENTS

INTRODUCTION 5

CHAPTER 1 9

Understanding Hypertension: Causes, Symptoms, and Risks 9

    The Question Now Is, What Brings on Hypertension? 11

    Signs And Symptoms of Hypertension 12

    Habits of daily life with high blood pressure: 14

    Conditions of the Body with High Blood Pressure: 15

    Alternative Methods of Treating Hypertension: 17

    Treatment and Management of Hypertension: 18

CHAPTER 2 21

Diagnosing Hypertension: Tests and Recommendations 21

    Diagnosing Hypertension: 21

    Exams to Determine Hypertension: 21

    Recommendations for Making a Diagnosis of High Blood Pressure: 22

    Hypertension May Lead to A Number of Complications. 24

    Managing Your Life with Hypertension: 29

    Alterations to One's Way of Life to Treat Hypertension: 30

CHAPTER 3 34

Lifestyle Changes for Hypertension Management: Diet, Exercise, and Stress Reduction 34

    Modifications to Your Diet 36

    Exercise 37

Stress Reduction 38

Further Suggestions That Can Assist You in Making Changes to Your Lifestyle That Will Last: 39

CHAPTER 4 42

Medications for Hypertension: Types, Dosages, and Side Effects 42

Some Of the Drugs for Hypertension That Are Used Most Frequently: 42

CHAPTER 5 49

Complementary and Alternative Therapies for Hypertension 49

CAM Therapy 49

Acupuncture 50

CHAPTER 6 58

Working with Your Healthcare Provider: Communication and Collaboration 58

Test Results 59

Record Keeping 60

CHAPTER 7 65

Staying Motivated and Adhering to Your Plan: Tips for Success, Overcoming Challenges and Maintaining Progress 65

Keeping Blood Pressure Under Control: 70

I. Keeping a Close Eye on Your Blood Pressure: 70

2. Modifying Your Current Course of Treatment: 71

3. Continuing in the Same Direction: 72

CONCLUSION 75

INTRODUCTION

Hypertension, often known as high blood pressure, is a prevalent medical condition that impacts the health of millions of individuals all over the globe. If hypertension is not managed, it may result in major health concerns such as heart disease, stroke, and kidney failure. The good news is that hypertension is a disease that can be managed, and with the correct attitude and assistance, it is possible to regulate your blood pressure and lower the risk of health issues that are associated with hypertension.

This book, Taking Control of Hypertension: A Comprehensive Guide to Lowering Your Blood Pressure, is intended to assist you in better understanding your condition and successfully managing it. This guide will offer you the knowledge, skills, and resources you need to take control of your health, regardless of whether or not you have just been diagnosed with hypertension or have been living with it for some time.

You will get an understanding of the conditions that may lead to hypertension, its symptoms, and the dangers that are associated with it, as well as the many therapies and adjustments to lifestyle that can help you control the disease. You will also be educated on the various drugs, complementary and alternative treatments, as well as the process of developing an individualized treatment plan in collaboration with your healthcare physician.

With the help of this book, you will be equipped with the information and self-assurance you need to take an active part in your healthcare and make the adjustments essential to achieving and maintaining control of your blood pressure. This handbook is an invaluable resource for anybody who wants to improve their overall health and well-being, whether their goal is to lower their risk of hypertension-related health issues or to simply enhance their general health.

This book will also cover the following topics in addition to the information and resources that were provided in the preceding introduction: • Understanding the many forms of hypertension and the causes of each type

• Determining the variables that put a person at risk for developing hypertension and taking measures to mitigate those risks.

• Analyze the behaviors you engage in daily and make adjustments to those behaviors to enhance your health and minimize stress.

• Investigating the many different drugs that may be used to control hypertension, including the advantages and disadvantages of each option.

• Investigating the potential benefits of complementary and alternative treatments, such as acupuncture, massage, and herbal medicines, for bringing down one's blood pressure.

• Being aware of how important it is to regularly monitor and record your blood pressure measurements, as well as how to understand the findings and take appropriate action based on them.

• Developing a specific action plan to assist you in achieving and maintaining control of your blood pressure, and defining objectives for your health and well-being that are both reasonable and attainable.

Taking Control of Hypertension: A Extensive Guide to Lowering Your Blood Pressure is a crucial resource for anybody who wants to take control of their hypertension and achieve greater health and well-being since it provides comprehensive coverage, practical guidance, and actionable ideas. This guide will help you negotiate the hurdles of managing your illness and empower you to take control of your health. Whether you have just been diagnosed with hypertension or have been living with it for years, this guide will help you take charge of your health.

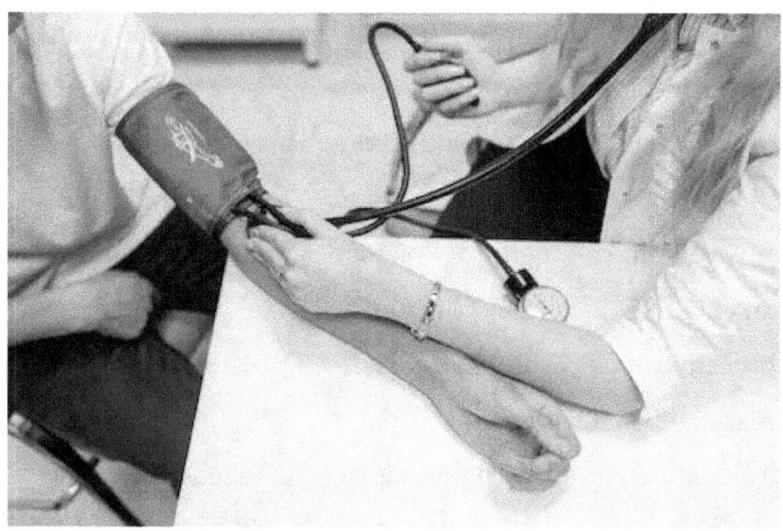

CHAPTER 1

Understanding Hypertension: Causes, Symptoms, and Risks

We are pleased to welcome you to the first section of our all-encompassing guide on bringing hypertension under control. In this chapter, we will investigate what hypertension, often known as high blood pressure, is as well as its causes, symptoms, and dangers that are associated with it.

First things first, let's take a moment to discuss what hypertension is. The disease known as hypertension occurs when the force of blood pushing against the walls of your arteries is regularly too high. This may, over time, cause damage to your blood vessels and raise your chance of developing heart disease, stroke, and other major health issues.

It is essential to keep in mind that not all of the elements that might lead to hypertension are within our control, despite the fact that there are numerous factors that can contribute to the condition. Age, the medical history of one's family, and one's race are all factors that could come into play. Because of this, it is very essential to place our attention on the aspects of our lives that are within our power to alter, such as the choices we make about our way of life, and to make an effort to reduce the likelihood that we may acquire hypertension.

When it comes to diagnosis, hypertension is generally considered to be present when your blood pressure readings routinely measure at a level that is higher than 140/90 mmHg. Because hypertension often does not exhibit any symptoms, it is important to get your blood pressure monitored on a regular basis. In addition to the checkups that are planned at regular intervals, your doctor may recommend that you monitor your blood pressure with a self-monitoring device while you are at home.

It is also necessary to have an understanding that there are several forms of hypertension, such as primary hypertension, which is sometimes referred to as essential hypertension, and secondary hypertension. Primary hypertension is the most prevalent form, and it is caused by an underlying mix of variables such as heredity, poor lifestyle behaviors, and other health disorders. Primary hypertension may lead to serious health complications. On the other hand, secondary hypertension is brought on by an underlying medical problem such as renal disease or sleep apnea. This kind of hypertension is more common in older adults.

What steps can you take to reduce your likelihood of getting high blood pressure, and how can you better manage your condition if you already have it? Making adjustments to your lifestyle, such as switching to a healthier diet, being more physically active on a regular basis, giving up smoking, and learning how to better manage stress, may have a beneficial effect on your blood pressure and general health. In addition, it is important to adhere to the treatment plan laid out by your physician and take your medicines exactly as directed in order to be successful in managing hypertension.

The Question Now Is, What Brings on Hypertension?

There is no one mechanism that leads to hypertension; rather, the illness is brought on by a confluence of variables, including heredity, bad lifestyle choices, and specific health problems. The following are some frequent causes:

• A diet that is not healthy: Heavy blood pressure may be caused or made worse by eating a diet that is high in salt, bad fats, and processed foods.

- Not getting enough exercise: Not moving around enough may contribute to weight gain and a sedentary lifestyle, both of which can raise blood pressure.
- Stress: Prolonged stress may contribute to higher-than-normal levels of blood pressure.
- Cigarette smoking: Cigarette smoking is a major risk factor for developing high blood pressure.
- Drinking an excessive amount of alcohol: Consuming an excessive amount of alcohol might lead to elevated blood pressure readings.

Signs And Symptoms of Hypertension

Now, let's have a look at the signs and symptoms of hypertension. The fact that many individuals who have hypertension do not feel any symptoms at all is one of the primary reasons why this condition is often known as the "silent killer." On the other hand, some individuals who have very high blood pressure may feel symptoms including headaches, dizziness, blurred vision, or discomfort in the chest.

It is also important to keep in mind that many behaviors that are part of a healthy lifestyle, such as consuming alcohol, might temporarily elevate your blood pressure. Even if it does not induce hypertension over the long term, consuming an excessive quantity of alcohol may cause damage to your blood vessels and raise your chance of developing heart disease, stroke, and other health complications.

Concerning the manifestations of hypertension, one must first be aware of the fact that not everyone who has the condition will show signs and symptoms of it. On the other hand, some individuals who have very high blood pressure may feel symptoms including headaches, dizziness, blurred vision, or discomfort in the chest. If you have any of these symptoms, it is imperative that you consult a medical professional as soon as possible since they may be indicators of a more severe problem.

It is essential that you have a solid understanding of the dangers associated with hypertension, since it may put you at an increased risk for a number of major health issues, including cardiovascular disease, stroke, renal disease, and loss of eyesight. It is also important to note that hypertension may be a contributing factor to other health issues, such as dementia and sexual dysfunction, and this is something that should be taken into consideration.

Furthermore, it is essential to have a solid understanding that hypertension may have a variety of distinct effects on certain populations. For instance, women who acquire hypertension during pregnancy, which is sometimes referred to as gestational hypertension, are at a greater risk of acquiring long-term hypertension in addition to other health issues. African Americans are also at a greater risk for hypertension as well as the health concerns that are often connected with it.

Persons who are overweight or obese, people who have a history of hypertension in their family, and people who are over the age of 65 are at an increased risk of developing hypertension. It is crucial to note that some groups are at an increased risk of developing hypertension.

Habits of daily life with high blood pressure:

Diet: An increased risk of hypertension may be associated with consuming a diet that is rich in sodium but low in potassium. Be aware of how much-processed food, fast food, and junk food you eat since these types of meals often contain a lot of salt. Consuming a diet that is abundant in fruits and vegetables, proteins that are low in fat, and whole grains may assist in the lowering of blood pressure.

Regular participation in physical activity has been shown to minimize the chance of acquiring hypertension as well as lower blood pressure in those who already have it. Aim to engage in some kind of moderately intense physical exercise for at least half an hour on most days of the week.

Cigarette smoking: Smoking is a significant risk factor for hypertension, in addition to being associated with a wide variety of other severe health issues. Stopping smoking is one of the most beneficial things you can do for your health if you are a smoker.

Conditions of the Body with High Blood Pressure:

Sleep apnea is a disorder that causes you to stop breathing during sleep, which may lead to an increase in blood pressure. Sleep apnea is also known as obstructive sleep apnea. If you have sleep apnea, getting treatment for it may help decrease your blood pressure and lessen the likelihood that you will develop hypertension.

Diabetes: High levels of blood sugar may cause damage to the blood vessels in your body, which might raise your chance of having high blood pressure (hypertension). Your chance of getting hypertension may be reduced as well as your blood pressure when you successfully manage your diabetes through a combination of diet, exercise, and medication.

Kidney disease: Kidney illness may cause damage to the blood vessels that are already present in your kidneys, which can contribute to high blood pressure. If you have kidney illness, having it diagnosed and treated as soon as possible will help decrease your blood pressure and lessen the likelihood that you will develop hypertension.

You are able to gain control of your blood pressure and lower the likelihood of developing major health issues by taking an active part in managing your health, which may include making adjustments to your lifestyle and taking care of any underlying medical concerns. Therefore, do not be afraid to communicate with your physician and ask them questions; they are there to assist you.

Alternative Methods of Treating Hypertension:

Alterations to one's lifestyle: Alterations to one's lifestyle, such as eating a better diet, increasing one's level of physical activity, giving up smoking, and taking steps to reduce stress, may all help decrease one's blood pressure.

Medication: If making adjustments to your lifestyle is not sufficient to regulate your blood pressure, your physician may prescribe medication to assist reduce it. Medication: Diuretics, angiotensin-converting enzyme (ACE) inhibitors, calcium channel blockers, and beta blockers are some of the different types of medications that can be used to treat hypertension. Monitoring: Regular monitoring of your blood pressure is an important part of the management of hypertension. It is possible that your physician may advise you to monitor your blood pressure either at home or in the office.

Working with your primary care provider to manage hypertension includes: Collaborating together with your healthcare provider to create a treatment strategy that is tailored specifically to your needs. You and your doctor will be able to establish whether or not your treatment plan is working well by keeping a close eye on your blood pressure and going in for regular checkups.

Take the initiative: Make an effort to improve your health by altering certain aspects of your lifestyle, such as keeping a close eye on your blood pressure and following the dosing instructions for any drugs that your doctor has given you.

Ask questions: Do not be scared to challenge your doctor; in fact, you should. They are there to assist you in the management of your health and provide answers to any queries you may have.

You may gain control of your blood pressure and lower your chance of developing major health issues by maintaining close communication with your primary care physician, making adjustments to your way of life, and taking any medicines that have been given to you. You can assist guarantee that you will continue to have healthy blood pressure for many years to come by implementing the appropriate treatment plan and monitoring it.

Treatment and Management of Hypertension:

Healthy lifestyle: Keeping a healthy lifestyle, which includes not smoking, getting regular physical activity, eating a healthy diet, and managing stress, can help prevent hypertension. Other components of a healthy lifestyle include: eating a healthy diet; getting regular physical activity; and eating regularly.

Managing your weight is an important part of hypertension prevention since being overweight or obese might raise your chance of having high blood pressure. Keeping your weight at a healthy level can help avoid hypertension.

Consuming an excessive quantity of alcohol may cause your blood pressure to rise. Because of this, it is imperative that you restrict the amount of alcohol you consume to no more than a drink each day for women and no more than two drinks each day for men.

Managing Your Life When You Have Hypertension • Know Your Numbers: Always keep a record of your blood pressure measurements and report any significant changes to your physician.

• Modify your lifestyle: To assist you in maintaining healthy blood pressure levels, you should modify aspects of your lifestyle such as the foods you consume, the amount of exercise you get, and the amount of stress you allow yourself to experience.

• Always follow the directions that come with your medication: Always follow your doctor's instructions while taking your blood pressure medicine, and never stop taking your prescription without first seeing your healthcare provider.

• Find healthy methods to handle stress, such as practicing relaxation techniques, engaging in physical activity, and spending time with loved ones; this will help you keep stress at bay.

Continue to see your primary care physician You should continue to see your primary care physician for follow-up visits on a regular basis so that he or she can help you monitor your blood pressure and alter your treatment plan as necessary.

If you follow these guidelines, you will be able to get your blood pressure under control, lower your chance of developing major health issues, and lead a lifestyle that is both healthy and active. Keep in mind that hypertension is a curable illness and that you may live a long and healthy life by following the recommended treatment plan and making adjustments to your lifestyle.

CHAPTER 2
Diagnosing Hypertension: Tests and Recommendations

Diagnosing Hypertension:

The first step in determining whether or not you have hypertension is to measure your blood pressure using a blood pressure cuff and write down the findings. A systolic blood pressure (the top number) of 140 or higher, or a diastolic blood pressure (the bottom number) of 90 or higher, is considered to be a diagnosis of high blood pressure. A physical examination and a review of your medical history may also be performed by your doctor in order to determine whether or not you have risk factors for developing hypertension. These risk factors can include your age, the history of hypertension in your family, and the lifestyle choices you make.

Exams to Determine Hypertension:

Your doctor will likely prescribe other tests in addition to testing your blood pressure in order to assist in the diagnosis of hypertension and discover the underlying cause of the condition. The following are examples of some of these examinations:

- Tests of your urine can determine whether or not you have protein or glucose in your urine, both of which may be signs of kidney disease.
- Cholesterol, glucose, and electrolyte levels in the blood will be measured at this step of the testing process.
- Electrocardiogram, sometimes known as an ECG, is a test that examines the electrical activity of your heart.
- Echocardiogram: This test evaluates the structure as well as the function of your heart.

Recommendations for Making a Diagnosis of High Blood Pressure:

Maintain a frequent check on your blood pressure: Maintaining a consistent monitoring schedule for your blood pressure may assist both you and your physician in determining whether or not you have hypertension and whether or not the medication is required.

- Check-in with your healthcare provider: Your doctor will be able to assist you to monitor your blood pressure and make any required adjustments to your treatment plan during your follow-up consultations at regular intervals.

- Notify your doctor of any symptoms: You should let your doctor know about any symptoms you may be having, including headaches, dizziness, or nosebleeds.
- Keep a record of what you have read: Always remember to record your blood pressure measurements and bring them with you when you see the doctor.

You can help ensure an accurate diagnosis of hypertension and receive the appropriate treatment to help control your blood pressure and reduce the risk of developing serious health problems by following these recommendations. You can also help ensure an accurate diagnosis of diabetes by following these recommendations. Keep in mind that getting an accurate diagnosis of your hypertension and beginning treatment as soon as possible is essential for preserving a healthy heart and lowering the likelihood of developing more significant health issues.

Hypertension May Lead to A Number of Complications.

If the condition is not addressed, hypertension may result in a variety of major health concerns, including the following:

Diseases of the heart: High blood pressure may cause damage to the blood vessels in your body, which in turn raises your chance of having a heart attack, stroke, or heart failure.

Kidney disease: High blood pressure may cause damage to your kidneys, which can lead to renal disease and ultimately kidney failure.

Eye damage: High blood pressure may cause the blood vessels in your eyes to get damaged, which can lead to a loss of vision.

Dementia: Having high blood pressure might make you more likely to acquire dementia, such as Alzheimer's disease.

Sexual dysfunction may be caused by high blood pressure, which can affect both men and women. Sexual dysfunction can occur in any gender.

It is essential to get a diagnosis of hypertension and begin treatment as soon as possible in order to lessen the likelihood of acquiring these major health concerns.

Modifications to Lifestyle and Medication Therapy for Hypertension: Modifications to lifestyle and medication therapy are often both components of hypertension treatment. Your physician could suggest that you take both of them together. The following modifications to your way of life may be suggested by your physician:

• Maintaining a healthy diet: Maintaining a nutritious diet that is low in salt, fat, and added sweets may assist in maintaining blood pressure regulation.

• Participating in regular physical exercise: Participating in regular physical activity may assist in lowering blood pressure and improving overall health.

• If you are overweight or obese, reducing the amount of weight you are carrying may assist in bringing down your blood pressure.

• Keeping your alcohol consumption to a reasonable level Because drinking an excessive quantity of alcohol may cause your blood pressure to rise, it is essential to keep your alcohol consumption to no more than one drink each day for women and no more than two drinks each day for men.

• Giving up smoking: Giving up smoking is one of the most important things you can do to enhance your health overall and decrease your blood pressure.

• Finding healthy methods to manage stress: Finding healthy ways to manage stress, such as practicing relaxation techniques, exercising, and spending time with loved ones, will help you keep a better handle on your blood pressure.

Medication for Hypertension: If your doctor diagnoses you with hypertension, he or she may prescribe medication to help you keep your blood pressure under control. The following are some of the most often-used drugs for hypertension:

- Diuretics are medications that assist your body get rid of extra fluid and salt, which in turn may bring your blood pressure down.
- ACE inhibitors assist relax your blood vessels and drop your blood pressure. ACE inhibitors are used in several hypertension medications.
- Calcium channel blockers Assist Relax Your Blood Vessels and Lower Your Blood Pressure Calcium

channel blockers help relax your blood vessels and lower your blood pressure.
- Beta-blockers are medications that lower blood pressure and heart rate. Beta-blockers also decrease your heart rate.
- Angiotensin receptor blockers, often known as ARBs, are a kind of medication that helps relax blood vessels and lower blood pressure.

You may help regulate your blood pressure and lower your chance of developing major health issues by making adjustments to your lifestyle and taking your medicines as advised. Keep in mind that hypertension is a curable illness, and if you choose the appropriate treatment plan, you may have a long and healthy life despite having hypertension.

Keeping an Eye on Your Blood Pressure After a diagnosis of hypertension has been made, it is essential to keep an eye on your blood pressure on a regular basis.

Your primary care physician would almost certainly advise you to have your blood pressure tested at least once a year, and maybe even more often if required. You may also check your blood pressure by utilizing a monitor that is designed specifically for use in the home. Keeping a record of your blood pressure might be particularly helpful in the intervals between appointments with the doctor.

If you are going to check your blood pressure at home, it is imperative that you use a blood pressure monitor that has been correctly calibrated and that you follow the instructions very carefully. In order to get the most reliable results from your blood pressure readings, you should try to take them at the same time each day, such as first thing in the morning and before bed.

If, after therapy, your blood pressure continues to be high, your physician may suggest that you undergo further testing to assist in determining the reason for your high blood pressure and to direct the treatment plan that is developed for you.

• Blood testing: Blood tests may help screen for underlying medical illnesses, such as renal disease or diabetes, that may be contributing to your high blood pressure. These tests may be performed if your doctor suspects that one of these diseases is the cause of your hypertension.

• A urinalysis is a test that may determine whether or not there is a protein in your urine, which is a sign that your kidneys may be damaged.

• Electrocardiogram (ECG): An ECG is a test that may assist determine whether or not a patient has heart disease, which is a typical consequence of hypertension.

Managing Your Life with Hypertension:

It may be difficult to live with hypertension, but if you find the correct treatment plan and make some adjustments to the way you live your life, you can get your blood pressure under control and lower your chance of developing significant health issues. The following are some of the methods that you may assist control your hypertension:

If you continue to follow your treatment plan: The key to successfully regulating your blood pressure is to take your medicines exactly as prescribed, make the modifications to your lifestyle that your doctor suggests, and test your blood pressure on a regular basis.

Talking to your doctor is essential if you want answers to any questions or concerns you have regarding your hypertension. If you have any questions or concerns, be sure to go to your doctor. They will be able to assist you in better understanding your situation and will provide you with the assistance that you need.

Modifying your lifestyle to make it healthier: quitting smoking, cutting back on alcohol consumption, adopting a healthier diet, increasing your level of regular physical activity, and developing strategies to deal with stress are all essential components of an effective hypertension management plan.

Maintaining an awareness of the most recent advancements in hypertension treatment will assist you in gaining a deeper understanding of your condition and enable you to make more educated choices about your medical care.

Keep in mind that hypertension is a curable illness, and if you choose the appropriate treatment plan, you may have a long and healthy life despite having hypertension. Do not be hesitant to speak to your doctor about the things that are concerning you and to seek their help and assistance as you make your way through this process.

Alterations to One's Way of Life to Treat Hypertension:

Alterations to one's way of life are an essential component of hypertension management and lowering one's vulnerability to the development of severe health issues.

Alterations to your lifestyle, such as those listed below, may have a role in lowering your blood pressure.

Eating a nutritious diet: Consuming a healthy diet that is abundant in fruits, vegetables, whole grains, and lean protein may assist in the lowering of blood pressure. Some particular dietary modifications that may be beneficial include lowering the amount of salt you consume, raising the amount of potassium you consume, and cutting down on the amount of alcohol you drink.

Participating in consistent physical activity: Your blood pressure may be lowered and your general health can improve by engaging in regular physical exercise, such as brisk walking, running, cycling, or swimming at a moderate to vigorous intensity. Aim to engage in some kind of moderately intense physical exercise for at least half an hour on most days of the week.

If you are overweight or obese, lowering your weight may help decrease your blood pressure. Losing weight can aid lower your blood pressure. Aim to lose weight in a steady and healthy way, such as by eating a balanced diet and obtaining regular physical exercise. This may be accomplished by setting a goal to lose weight in this manner.

Putting an end to one's smoking habit: Smoking is a significant risk factor for high blood pressure as well as a wide variety of other health issues. Stopping smoking is one of the most beneficial things you can do for your health if you are a smoker.

Managing stress: Because prolonged stress may cause an increase in blood pressure, it is essential to find healthy strategies to handle stress, such as meditating, practicing deep breathing, or engaging in physical activity.

Your physician will collaborate with you to come up with the most effective treatment strategy for your hypertension, taking into consideration the specific requirements of your case as well as your past medical history.

Keep in mind that it is essential to take your meds exactly as prescribed and to adhere very completely to the treatment plan that has been laid out for you. Make sure to see your physician if you have any inquiries or concerns about the medicines you are taking. They will be able to assist you in better understanding your situation and will provide you with the assistance that you need.

CHAPTER 3
Lifestyle Changes for Hypertension Management: Diet, Exercise, and Stress Reduction

The most crucial preventable contributor to cardiovascular disease and death is high blood pressure, sometimes known as hypertension. Children who consume a lot of salt may be more likely to develop hypertension in adulthood.

Even a little reduction in the amount of salt consumed by people all over the globe would have a significant impact on improving public health. In relation to smoking as an additional risk factor, there are many different approaches that may be taken to encourage people to give up the habit. It is in the best interest of patients to have their physicians assist them in quitting smoking.

When it comes to the prevention of hypertension, a strategy that focuses on certain segments of the population may prove to be more beneficial than one that targets the community as a whole. It is highly suggested that one consumes a diet that is abundant in fruits and vegetables that are high in potassium.

The usual potassium level of meals is lowered when they are canned or frozen, thus the ideal items are fresh ones. Calcium supplementation lowers blood pressure in hypertensive people during chronic nitric oxide synthase suppression, and a high calcium diet improves vasorelaxation in nitric oxide-deficient hypertension. Anyone interested in lowering their risk of developing high blood pressure or treating it should give magnesium some consideration.

A balanced diet, regular exercise, stress reduction, and proper levels of potassium and magnesium serve as the basis for good blood pressure; nevertheless, further research is necessary before providing conclusive therapeutic recommendations on the usage of magnesium. Drinking alcohol is a factor in the development of hypertension that is often overlooked by medical professionals.

Stress management could be regarded as a potential solution for hypertension individuals in whom it seems that stress is a significant concern. It is more probable that individualized cognitive behavioral therapies will be beneficial than interventions consisting of a single component.

Modifications to Your Diet

Making changes to your diet is one of the most important things you can do to control your hypertension and lower your chance of developing major health issues. The following are some alterations to one's diet that may be helpful:

Reduce the amount of salt you consume. Consuming an excessive amount of salt may cause your body to retain fluid, which can lead to an increase in blood pressure. If you already have high blood pressure, you should strive for a salt intake that is even lower than the recommended daily maximum of 2,300 milligrams and try to keep your salt consumption at that level.

Your blood pressure may be lowered and the effects of sodium can be mitigated if you consume more potassium. Potassium can help offset the effects of sodium. Fruits and vegetables such as bananas, oranges, cantaloupe, strawberries, and leafy greens are all excellent providers of the mineral potassium.

Consume a diet that is abundant in fruit and vegetables: Because of their high vitamin content and low salt content, fruits and vegetables are excellent additions to a diet that is focused on health. Make it a daily goal to consume at least five servings worth of fruits and veggies.

Pick a protein that is low in fat: You may make yourself feel full and content while keeping your calorie consumption in control by eating lean proteins like chicken, fish, or tofu. These foods can help you keep your weight in check as well. Consume alcohol in moderation Since drinking an excessive amount of alcohol might cause your blood pressure to rise, it is essential to keep your alcohol consumption to no more than one drink per day for women and no more than two drinks per day for men.

Exercise

The treatment of hypertension and maintenance of general good health both depend heavily on regular physical activity, namely exercise. Here are some recommendations to help you get started:

Aim to engage in some kind of moderately intense physical exercise for at least half an hour on most days of the week.

This might involve sports such as running, cycling, swimming, or even just brisk walking at a fast pace. Your level of physical activity should, over time, progressively increase both in terms of its length and its intensity. Mix it up! Experiment with a wide variety of sports and workouts to maintain your interest and keep things fresh.

Include some kind of physical exercise in each day of your regimen. For instance, you may go for a stroll during your lunch break or ride your bike after supper to get some exercise.

Stress Reduction

Reducing Stress Because prolonged stress may cause an increase in blood pressure, it is essential to learn how to deal with stress in a healthy manner. The following is a list of approaches for stress reduction that you may find helpful:

Meditation: Meditation has been shown to reduce emotions of stress and anxiety by helping people relax and concentrate their minds.

Deep Breathing: In order to alleviate emotions of tension and worry, practicing deep breathing may assist reduce your heart rate and bring about a state of mental calmness.

Physical activity: Physical activity is an excellent strategy to lower stress levels and enhance overall health.

Get enough rest: Getting an adequate amount of sleep is critical for effective stress management and for sustaining excellent health. Aim to get between 7 and 9 hours of sleep per night.

Altering one's way of life may be a significant obstacle, but it is essential to keep in mind that one does not have to make all of the necessary adjustments at once. Begin with adjustments that are easily controllable and progressively work your way up from there. Also, don't forget to acknowledge the positive improvements you have brought about in yourself! Each movement in the correct direction is a step toward improved physical well-being.

Further Suggestions That Can Assist You in Making Changes to Your Lifestyle That Will Last:

Find a network of people to lean on: Finding people in your life — whether they be friends, family, or members of a support group — who are on board with the changes you want to make in your lifestyle and who provide encouragement may be a tremendous asset.

Establish objectives that can be attained: Keeping yourself motivated and on track may be made easier if you establish goals that are both practical and attainable. For instance, if you want to increase the amount of physical activity you do, you might begin by making it a goal to walk for ten minutes every day, and then over time, you could progressively increase both the length and the intensity of your walks.

Keep a record of what you eat: Keeping a food diary may assist you in being more aware of what you are consuming and can make it simpler to pinpoint specific areas in which you can improve your diet and eating habits.

Make it fun: Including regular exercise and nutritious eating as part of your daily routine may make these activities more pleasurable if you make them fun for yourself. In order to maintain your motivation, you may try out some new recipes, sign up for a sports team, or look for a workout partner.

Give yourself a treat: Honor the milestones of your progress along the journey! When you hit a key milestone or make a substantial adjustment to your lifestyle, you should celebrate the accomplishment by treating yourself to a reward of some kind, such as a massage or a new book.

Making adjustments to one's way of life may be challenging, but the positive effects on one's health and well-being make the effort worthwhile. You are able to accomplish your objectives and regain control of your hypertension if you have a good attitude and are persistent.

CHAPTER 4
Medications for Hypertension: Types, Dosages, and Side Effects

Many individuals who have high blood pressure depend on medication to help them keep their condition under control since the medication is an essential component in the management of hypertension (also known as high blood pressure). There are many various kinds of drugs that may be used to treat hypertension, and each one acts in a somewhat different manner to bring the patient's blood pressure down.

Some Of the Drugs for Hypertension That Are Used Most Frequently:

Inhibitors of the enzyme angiotensin-converting enzyme (ACE): ACE inhibitors function by relaxing the blood arteries, which results in increased blood flow and a reduction in the amount of pressure that is placed on the heart. People who suffer from hypertension as well as other health concerns, such as heart disease or diabetes, often get prescriptions for this category of drug. Lisinopril, enalapril, and ramipril are a few examples of medications that fall under the category of ACE inhibitors.

Angiotensin Receptor Blockers (ARBs): ARBs are similar to ACE inhibitors, but they work by blocking the effects of angiotensin, which is a hormone that causes blood vessels to narrow and raises blood pressure. ACE inhibitors work by inhibiting the production of renin, which is a protein that causes blood vessels to widen. People who are unable to take ACE inhibitors owing to the potential for adverse effects or for other reasons may be given ARBs as an alternative treatment. Examples of ARBs are losartan, valsartan, and irbesartan.

Calcium Channel Blockers (CCBs): CCBs function by relaxing the blood vessels and lessening the power of the heart's contractions. Calcium channel blockers are also known as calcium channel antagonists. People who suffer from hypertension as well as other health conditions, such as heart disease or angina, often get prescriptions for this category of drug. The medications amlodipine, nifedipine, and diltiazem are all examples of CCBs.

Diuretics are a kind of medication that is often provided to patients in order to assist them in managing their hypertension. These medications are effective because they rid the body of extra fluid, which in turn lowers the volume of blood and the pressure that is placed on the heart. The medications hydrochlorothiazide, furosemide, and chlorthalidone are all considered to be diuretics.

Beta-blockers: Beta-blockers decrease the heart rate and reduce the power of the heart's contractions in order to achieve their therapeutic effect. People who suffer from hypertension as well as other health conditions, such as heart disease or angina, often get prescriptions for this category of drug. Metoprolol, atenolol, and propranolol are a few examples of medications that are classified as beta blockers. It is essential to take your prescriptions in the manner prescribed by your medical professional. This includes taking the prescribed dosage at the prescribed time as well as adhering to any additional instructions, such as whether or not the drug should be taken with or without meals. If you have any concerns about your prescriptions, whether they be side effects or interactions with other drugs, it is essential to discuss these issues with your primary care physician.

Drugs used to treat hypertension might have adverse effects, just like any other treatment. The following are some of the adverse effects of hypertension medication that are most often experienced:

- Cough
- Headache
- Nausea or vomiting
- Diarrhea or constipation
- Weakness or tiredness
- Swelling or fluid retention
- Chest discomfort or heart palpitations
- Lightheadedness or dizziness
- Cough • Headache
- Nausea or vomiting
- Diarrhea or constipation
- Weakness or fatigue

These negative effects are often not severe and typically disappear within a few days to a few weeks. On the other hand, some individuals can develop more severe adverse effects, such as a racing pulse, chest discomfort, or trouble breathing. If you encounter any of these side effects, you should immediately stop taking the medicine and make an appointment with your primary care physician.

It's possible that the painkillers, birth control pills, or antifungal treatments you're taking could react negatively with the hypertension medication you're taking in some circumstances. It is imperative that you inform your primary care physician about all of the prescriptions you are currently taking, including any over-the-counter meds, in order for them to do any necessary drug interaction checks.

It is essential to keep in mind that hypertension is a chronic ailment and that treating it calls for a dedication that lasts a person's whole life. It is possible that medications on their own may not be sufficient to adequately manage your blood pressure, and that adjustments to your lifestyle will need to be modified as necessary over time. Maintaining consistent monitoring and adjustment of your medicines, in addition to maintaining a solid working relationship with your primary care physician, is crucial in order to guarantee that your hypertension is well controlled.

In addition, it is essential to be knowledgeable about the possibility of adverse drug interactions and to disclose to your physician any other drugs that you are currently taking. Certain drugs have the potential to interact with one another in a way that may either increase or diminish the efficacy of either of the medications. Alcohol, for instance, may produce low blood pressure and interact negatively with some blood pressure medicines, while nonsteroidal anti-inflammatory drugs (NSAIDs) can raise blood pressure and reduce the efficacy of blood pressure medications.

It is also essential to be aware of any symptoms that may suggest that your blood pressure is not being properly regulated. Some of these symptoms include headaches, dizziness, chest discomfort, shortness of breath, and changes in vision. It is imperative that you schedule an appointment with your primary care physician as soon as possible if you encounter any of these symptoms. Uncontrolled hypertension may lead to a variety of significant health issues, including heart disease, stroke, and damage to the kidneys.

In conclusion, the management of hypertension entails making adjustments to one's lifestyle, undergoing frequent monitoring, and taking drugs in the manner that has been recommended. You may establish a comprehensive strategy to properly regulate your blood pressure, lower the risk of significant health issues, and improve your overall health and quality of life with the assistance of your doctor.

CHAPTER 5

Complementary and Alternative Therapies for Hypertension

Complementary and alternative therapies for hypertension, commonly known as CAM therapies, are a variety of treatments and techniques that are used in combination with traditional medical treatments for hypertension or as an alternative to such treatments.

Despite the fact that these therapies are not typically regarded as viable alternatives to the tried-and-true medical treatments for hypertension, a significant number of individuals who have high blood pressure turn to them as a method to control their disease and enhance their overall health.

CAM Therapy

Relaxation and stress reduction practices including deep breathing, meditation, and yoga are examples of some of the most popular complementary and alternative medicine (CAM) treatments for hypertension. The use of these approaches has been demonstrated to have a beneficial impact on one's blood pressure levels, as well as a beneficial impact on one's ability to alleviate stress, which is a key contributor to high blood pressure.

Garlic, coenzyme Q10, and magnesium are just a few examples of herbal supplements that are often used to treat and control hypertension.

Even if it has been shown that some of these supplements have a moderate influence on the levels of blood pressure, it is essential to exercise extreme caution while taking them since they may mix with other drugs and have the potential to cause negative effects. It is important that you discuss any herbal supplement you are considering taking with your primary care provider first to evaluate whether or not it will be beneficial to you.

Acupuncture

Another complementary and alternative medicine treatment that is occasionally used to control hypertension is acupuncture, which is a kind of traditional Chinese medicine. Acupuncture is a kind of treatment in which very thin needles are inserted into particular sites on the body.

The goals of this treatment are to enhance blood flow, promote relaxation, and lower levels of stress. There is some evidence to indicate that acupuncture may be useful in decreasing the levels of blood pressure; however, further study is required to establish both the efficacy and safety of acupuncture for this usage.

Finally, omega-3 fatty acids and the DASH diet are two examples of nutritional supplements that are often utilized as supplemental therapy for hypertension. It has been shown that following a DASH diet, which emphasizes eating a lot of fruits, vegetables, whole grains, and low-fat dairy products, will successfully bring blood pressure readings down. It has also been proven that omega-3 fatty acids, which may be found in fish as well as in certain plant-based diets, can have a beneficial influence on the levels of blood pressure.

In addition, while complementary and alternative medicine (CAM) treatments for hypertension may be a helpful adjunct to standard medical treatments for the condition, it is essential to exercise caution and have enough information before utilizing them. Before beginning treatment with any complementary and alternative medicine (CAM), it is critical to discuss the matter with your primary care provider to ascertain whether the treatment will be risk-free and suitable for you, as well as to ensure that your hypertension will be effectively controlled. Keep in mind that your health is a journey, and the key to successfully managing your blood pressure and improving your overall health and quality of life is to work with your doctor to find the right combination of treatments and approaches that work best for you. This is the key to successfully managing your blood pressure.

There are a number of other complementary methods that have been used for the management of hypertension in addition to the CAM treatments that were discussed before. Some examples of this are as follows:

Massage treatment: Massage therapy may assist to lessen stress levels and increase circulation, both of which can contribute to a reduction in blood pressure levels. Regular massage treatment may help to improve relaxation and decrease feelings of anxiety, both of which can contribute to high blood pressure. This can be helpful in reducing the risk of developing high blood pressure.

Adjustments made to the spine and joints during chiropractic therapy may assist to enhance the function of the nervous system and induce relaxation. Chiropractic care also includes the manipulation of the spine and joints. There is a need for further study in this field, despite the fact that certain studies have shown evidence that chiropractic treatment may be useful in lowering blood pressure.

Homeopathic treatments include: Homeopathic treatments are administered by using very diluted versions of naturally occurring compounds in order to encourage the body's natural healing response. These treatments are predicated on the theory that "like heals like." Some individuals feel that using homeopathic treatments for hypertension is beneficial in regulating their blood pressure, despite the fact that there is minimal scientific evidence to support the use of homeopathic medicines for the condition.

Biofeedback is a method that includes monitoring and delivering feedback on a number of different physiological processes. Some examples of these functions are heart rate and blood pressure. Individuals may learn how to manage and regulate these processes with the aid of this feedback, which may also be helpful in lowering stress and worry, two factors that can lead to high blood pressure.

Aromatherapy: Aromatherapy is the practice of using essential oils, such as lavender and chamomile, to facilitate a state of relaxation and cut down on feelings of anxiety and tension. Although there is still a need for more study to be done in this area, there is evidence from a few studies that suggests that the usage of essential oils may assist to decrease the levels of blood pressure.

It is essential to keep in mind that certain complementary and alternative medicine (CAM) treatments may be risk-free and useful for the management of hypertension, whilst other CAM therapies may cause damage or interact negatively with traditional medical treatments. Always have a discussion with your primary care provider before beginning any complementary and alternative medicine (CAM) treatment to confirm that the treatment will be safe and effective for you.

Managing hypertension, on the other hand, may be done using a variety of treatments that fall under the umbrella of complementary and alternative medicine. It is important to be informed and cautious when using any of these therapies and to consult with your doctor to determine whether or not they are safe and appropriate for you.

Even though some of these therapies may be effective in lowering blood pressure levels, it is still important to be informed about them. It is important to keep in mind that your health is a journey, and the best way to successfully manage your blood pressure and improve your overall health and quality of life is to work with your doctor to find the right combination of treatments and approaches that work best for you. Working together with your doctor is the key to successfully managing your blood pressure.

It is essential to bear in mind that complementary and alternative medicine (CAM) treatments for hypertension should in no way be seen as a replacement for standard medical therapy. Although there is some evidence that complementary and alternative medicine (CAM) treatments may be helpful in lowering blood pressure, it is recommended that these treatments be used in combination with traditional medical practices and lifestyle adjustments to get the best possible outcomes. In addition, it is essential to keep in mind that certain complementary and alternative medicine (CAM) treatments may have potential adverse effects, may interact negatively with traditional medical therapy, and may not be appropriate or safe for all patients. Before beginning treatment with any kind of complementary and alternative medicine (CAM), it is important to check in with your primary care provider to be sure that the treatment will be both safe and effective for you.

When reviewing the evidence for complementary and alternative medicine (CAM) treatments, it is essential to have both an educated and critical mindset. Although the results of a few studies could indicate that a certain complementary and alternative medicine (CAM) treatment is useful for the management of hypertension, these results need to be confirmed by further research that is rigorous and well-designed. Always check with your primary care physician before attempting anything new, and be aware of over-the-counter goods and therapies that make exaggerated or unfounded claims about their potential to decrease blood pressure.

When it comes to the management of hypertension, complementary and alternative medicine (CAM) treatments may be an effective addition to traditional medical treatments and changes in lifestyle. However, it is essential to approach complementary and alternative medicine (CAM) treatments with care and to always speak with a doctor in order to verify that they are both safe and effective. It is important to keep in mind that the most successful method for the management of hypertension is a combination of alterations to one's lifestyle, conventional medical treatments, and, if appropriate, complementary therapies undertaken under the supervision of a qualified healthcare professional.

Before beginning any complementary and alternative medicine treatment, it is important to have a conversation with your primary care physician or another qualified medical professional. In addition, it is essential to keep in mind that complementary and alternative medicine (CAM) treatments are not an alternative to traditional medical treatments, nor should they be utilized in lieu of changes to one's lifestyle or prescription medication. Alternative and complementary medicine (CAM) treatments have the potential to enhance overall heart health and bring blood pressure down when used in conjunction with the right kind of advice and monitoring.

CHAPTER 6

Working with Your Healthcare Provider: Communication and Collaboration

It is essential to have a solid working relationship with your healthcare practitioner in order to successfully manage hypertension. They are able to guide you through the process of making adjustments to your lifestyle, medicines, and other therapies, as well as track your progress over time. To get the most out of this partnership, however, it is essential to communicate in an open and efficient manner and to play an active role in your own care. Only then will you be able to realize the full potential of this relationship.

You should bring a list of questions and concerns with you to your meeting since this is one of the first things you can do. You may increase the likelihood of having a fruitful discussion and obtaining all of the information you need by doing this. You may also find it helpful to bring a close friend or member of your family along for added support.

It is essential that you communicate openly and honestly with your healthcare practitioner about any changes to your lifestyle as well as any drugs you may be taking. This covers drugs that may be purchased without a prescription, herbal supplements, and other forms of treatment. Your healthcare practitioner will be able to assist you in determining whether or not these items are safe and suitable for you, as well as whether or not your treatment plan should be adjusted appropriately.

Test Results

Understanding both your test findings and your diagnosis is another essential part of engaging with the healthcare physician who is responsible for your treatment. Be careful to inquire about the meaning of your blood pressure readings, as well as the findings of any other tests, and what they imply for your overall health. You should also inquire about the advantages and disadvantages of the various treatment choices, as well as what you should anticipate in terms of the short-term and long-term consequences of the therapy.

In addition, it is essential to work with your healthcare practitioner to build a treatment strategy that takes into account frequent checkups, adjustments to your way of life, and any drugs or therapies that you may need. If you have a detailed strategy, it will be easier for you to maintain your motivation and keep on track, and it will also give a framework for tracking how far you've come over time.

Record Keeping

It is recommended that you maintain a record of your blood pressure measurements, any symptoms you may encounter, and any modifications to your treatment plan or lifestyle that you make. This may assist you in recognizing patterns and trends over time, and it can offer your healthcare provider crucial information when you tend to visit them.

In addition to this, it is essential that you educate yourself about hypertension and the treatment choices that are available to you. Read patient resources such as books, articles, and other reading material, and think about joining a support group. This may help you understand your illness better and give you a stronger sense of control over your treatment.

It is essential that you acknowledge the possibility that, despite the modifications to your lifestyle and the adherence to your treatment plan, there may be occasions when your blood pressure does not react as favorably as you had anticipated it would. Do not get disheartened; rather, discuss with your healthcare physician the possibility of modifying your strategy or experimenting with other methods.

In addition to that, don't discount the significance of taking care of yourself. Keeping hypertension under control may be a commitment for a long period of time; thus, it is essential to take care of yourself on both a physical and an emotional level. Be sure to make getting enough sleep, managing your stress, exercising, and eating well your top priorities, and if you find yourself in need of help, don't hesitate to call out to friends, family, or a mental health professional.

Additionally, it is essential to have an open and honest line of communication with your healthcare practitioner. Inform your healthcare practitioner if you are having any uncomfortable side effects while taking your drugs or if you are not taking them as directed. You will be able to identify solutions that work for you and that will assist you in reaching your blood pressure objectives if you collaborate with one another.

In addition, it is beneficial to have open communication about any issues or questions you may have about the treatment plan you are following. For instance, if you are concerned about the expense of your drugs or the possibility of them causing you to have adverse effects, discuss these things with your healthcare professional. Your healthcare practitioner is in the best position to offer you the information and support you need to make educated choices about your treatment.

Do not be hesitant to get a second opinion if you are not feeling happy with the treatment plan that you are currently following or if you are not experiencing the outcomes that you had hoped for. Your health should be your number one concern, and getting a second opinion will help you determine whether or not you are receiving the finest treatment available.

In addition to that, take charge of your health management. Record the readings taken of your blood pressure, take note of any symptoms you may be experiencing, and schedule follow-up visits with your healthcare provider on a consistent basis so they can track your improvement. This might assist in guaranteeing that you remain on track and continue to make progress toward the objectives you have set for yourself.

In addition to this, it is essential to keep up to date on the most recent management strategies, medications, and developments in the field of hypertension. This information may assist you in having educated talks with your healthcare practitioner as well as in making informed choices about your treatment.

For instance, there are new pharmaceuticals under development that may have fewer adverse effects, and there are also new technologies such as wearable devices that can track and monitor your blood pressure continually. Both of these examples are examples of medical advancements. It is essential that you remain current on these breakthroughs and have a conversation about them with your healthcare physician in order to determine whether or not they may be of use to you.

Understanding the findings of any diagnostic tests or laboratory work that you have already submitted yourself to is also an essential part of working with your chosen healthcare practitioner. You should ask your provider to explain the findings and what they signify for your health, and you should be sure to ask any questions that come to mind.

Last but not least, it is essential that you have an understanding of the role that other medical experts may play in your treatment. You may work with a team of physicians, including a primary care physician, a specialist such as a cardiologist, and a pharmacist, depending on your unique requirements and the treatment plan that has been devised for you. This healthcare team is able to give you complete treatment and assistance to assist you in managing your hypertension because they collaborate closely together. In conclusion, cooperating with your healthcare practitioner calls for proactive communication, the making of well-informed decisions, and a desire to search for the most recent therapies and breakthroughs in the field. You can guarantee that you are getting the best possible care to manage your hypertension and improve your overall health and well-being by following these steps, which will allow you to ensure that you are receiving the best possible treatment.

CHAPTER 7

Staying Motivated and Adhering to Your Plan: Tips for Success, Overcoming Challenges and Maintaining Progress

Maintaining your motivation and sticking to your hypertension management plan might be difficult, but it is very necessary if you want to keep your health in excellent shape and steer clear of the major health problems that are linked with high blood pressure. The following are some suggestions for achieving success, prevailing over obstacles, and making consistent development.

Establish objectives that can be accomplished: Collaborate with your healthcare practitioner to establish objectives that are both attainable and reasonable for bringing your blood pressure under control. You may get closer to achieving your objectives by frequently monitoring your blood pressure at home, making any necessary adjustments to your medicines, maintaining a healthy diet, and engaging in regular physical activity.

Keep an eye on how far you've come: Keeping a record of your progress will help you recognize how far you've come and keep you inspired to continue moving forward with your goals. Record your blood pressure measurements, the drugs you take, and the modifications you make to your lifestyle, and then follow your improvement over time.

Put yourself in a position where you are surrounded by support: Having a solid support system may assist you in remaining on track and motivated. Discuss your objectives with members of your family and circle of friends, and look for support from those who have been successful in bringing their hypertension under control.

Maintaining a regular exercise routine is an essential component in the process of hypertension management. Participating in routine physical activity, such as walking, running, cycling, or swimming, may assist in the lowering of blood pressure and the improvement of general health.

It is crucial to identify healthy methods to manage stress since stress may have a detrimental influence on blood pressure. As a result, it is necessary to manage stress in a healthy manner. Think about trying out some mindfulness meditation, deep breathing, or yoga if you want to learn how to deal better with stress and enhance your general health.

Maintain your involvement: Maintaining your involvement in your own health and well-being might assist you in remaining motivated and on track. Attend support group meetings, study books and articles pertaining to hypertension, and become involved in community activities that are linked to the condition.

Reward yourself: Rewards are a terrific way to remain motivated and celebrate your accomplishments, and rewarding yourself is a great way to do both. After you have accomplished a certain objective, you should give some thought to rewarding yourself with something that you take pleasure in doing, such as getting a massage or spending the evening with your friends.

Maintain your ability to adapt because of the unpredictability of life and the fact that it may be impossible to always keep to your strategy. Maintain a flexible attitude and give yourself permission to make adjustments to your strategy when circumstances warrant. If you make a mistake, rather than berating yourself for it, try to get back on track as quickly as you can.

Conquer obstacles: Keeping hypertension under control is a process that lasts a lifetime, and there are certain to be obstacles along the road. The important thing is to figure out what the obstacles are and how to get around them. Collaborate with your healthcare practitioner to address any challenges you may be facing, and reach out to loved ones and friends for support when you need it.

Sure! When it comes to keeping up with your strategy and continuing to make progress, having a solid support system is essential. This might come from people you already know, such as friends and relatives, or through a support group designed exclusively for people who have hypertension. The motivation and direction you need to succeed might come from the support of others.

Setting objectives for yourself that are attainable and keeping track of your accomplishments along the way is also very essential. Motivating yourself to continue working toward your goals by noting and celebrating even the smallest achievements may be a big benefit.

Nevertheless, it is to be expected that there would be difficulties and impediments along the path. It is essential to not be too harsh on yourself and to make sure that you have a strategy in place for when something like this occurs. For instance, if you make a mistake and consume items that are bad for you, you shouldn't be too hard on yourself about it. Instead, make it your priority to get back on track with the next meal you eat or the activity you do.

Another piece of advice is to maintain a sense of variety and excitement throughout the process. This might be as easy as trying a new meal that is good for you or attempting a new kind of exercise. The ability to switch things up might help keep you interested and stave off boredom.

In addition to this, it is critical to maintain a feeling of responsibility and to keep oneself responsible. This might include working together with a friend or a healthcare practitioner to hold each other responsible, or it could involve locating an accountability partner via a support group.

Keep in mind that controlling hypertension is a journey that lasts a lifetime, and there will be both highs and lows along the road. The secret is to maintain a good attitude, maintain a focus on making progress, and resist the urge to give up when presented with obstacles.

Keeping Blood Pressure Under Control:

Keeping an Eye on It, Making Any Necessary Changes, and Sticking to Your Routine

I. Keeping a Close Eye on Your Blood Pressure:

A. Maintaining a Regular Checkup Schedule It is essential to maintain a regular checkup schedule with your healthcare provider in order to monitor your blood pressure and ensure that it remains within a healthy range. This should be done anywhere between once every three months and once every month if your blood pressure is not under good control.

B. Monitoring at Home: In addition to having their blood pressure checked at regular intervals, many individuals who have hypertension find that monitoring their blood pressure at home is beneficial. This enables you to monitor how changes in your lifestyle and medication affect your blood pressure and to track any swings that may occur as a result of those changes.

C. Monitoring Your Progress: Keeping a journal of your blood pressure measurements, including readings taken at home as well as readings taken at the office of your healthcare provider, will assist you in recognizing recurring patterns and trends over the course of time. You and your healthcare practitioner may use this information to make more educated choices about how to alter your treatment plan as a result.

2. Modifying Your Current Course of Treatment:

A. Modifications to Your Lifestyle Modifying your eating habits, your exercise regimen, and the ways in which you deal with stress may have a significant effect on your blood pressure. If you are having trouble keeping your blood pressure under control, your healthcare practitioner may suggest that you make further adjustments to your lifestyle, such as cutting down on the amount of salt you consume or giving up smoking.

B. Alterations to Medication In the event that making adjustments to your lifestyle alone are not sufficient to bring your blood pressure under control, your healthcare practitioner may make alterations to your medicines or add additional drugs to your treatment plan. It is essential to have a solid working relationship with your healthcare practitioner in order to determine the optimal mix of drugs and doses for your specific needs.

C. Keeping Track of Any Potential Adverse Effects It is essential that you keep track of any potential adverse effects that may be caused by the medications you are taking and communicate this information to your healthcare practitioner. They may be able to alter your doses or drugs in such a way as to reduce the severity of any adverse effects while maintaining an adequate level of blood pressure management.

3. Continuing in the Same Direction:

A. Adherence to the Treatment Plan In order to keep your blood pressure under control, you need to stick to your treatment plan on a continuous basis. This plan may include changes to your lifestyle as well as drugs. If you want to improve your health and lower your risk of hypertension-related issues, it is absolutely necessary for you to make substantial adjustments to your typical daily activities.

B. Coping with Setbacks: It is natural to have setbacks while you are attempting to regulate your blood pressure; nonetheless, it is crucial to stay the course and not give up on your efforts. Collaborate together with your healthcare practitioner to identify potential answers and discuss any necessary modifications to your treatment plan.

C. Commemorating Successes: Commemorating your successes along the road, such as meeting a new blood pressure target or successfully adhering to an adjustment to your lifestyle that is intended to make you healthier, may help you stay motivated and on track.

In conclusion, if you want to avoid the major health repercussions that are linked with high blood pressure, it is crucial that you keep your motivation and adhere to the hypertension treatment strategy that you have created for yourself. You can successfully manage your hypertension and keep your health in good shape by providing yourself with support, tracking your progress, setting reasonable goals, seeking support, remaining active, effectively managing stress, remaining engaged, rewarding yourself, being flexible, and overcoming challenges.

CONCLUSION

Keeping hypertension under control is one of the most important things you can do to protect your health and lower your chance of developing significant health issues. The first step in regaining control of your hypertension is gaining an understanding of its origins, symptoms, and associated dangers.

It is essential to have a correct diagnosis before deciding on the most appropriate treatment, which may be accomplished via testing and the advice of a healthcare expert. Alterations to one's lifestyle, including one's eating habits, level of physical activity, and level of stress, are just as important in the management of hypertension as the use of pharmaceuticals and complementary and alternative treatments. It is essential to maintain clear and efficient communication with your healthcare practitioner, to check your progress on a frequent basis, and to retain your motivation to stick to your treatment plan. You may take charge of your health and lower the likelihood of experiencing major health issues if you follow a holistic approach to controlling hypertension (also known as hypertension management).

In addition, it is essential to keep in mind that treating hypertension is an ongoing process rather than a simple problem that can be solved once and for all. You can assist guarantee that your success will continue by checking it on a regular basis and making any required modifications to your lifestyle and pharmaceutical regimen. A major difference may also be made in establishing and keeping control of one's blood pressure by maintaining one's motivation and dedication to one's strategy, as well as by seeking help when it is required.

The advantages of better health and a lower risk of significant health issues are worth the work of taking control of hypertension, which needs effort, dedication, and a good attitude. In general, however, taking control of hypertension requires effort. Managing hypertension is a challenge that, if faced with the appropriate information, tools, and resources, can be surmounted, resulting in a life that is both healthier and more fulfilling.

Additionally, it is essential to be knowledgeable about the possible adverse effects of drugs and to inform your healthcare practitioner of any symptoms that are out of the ordinary. Keeping up with your provider at regular intervals will assist verify that your treatment plan is still producing the desired results and that any required modifications are being made. Monitoring your blood pressure on a consistent basis, both at home and at visits may help you and your healthcare provider track your progress and make any required changes to your treatment plan. This monitoring can be done both at home and during appointments. In addition, leading a healthy lifestyle, which includes engaging in regular physical activity, consuming a diet that is both nutritionally and emotionally satisfying, and practicing techniques to reduce stress can help improve overall health and well-being, in addition to making it easier to regulate blood pressure.

Taking Control of Your Hypertension is a Step-by-Step Guide That Will Help You Lower Your Blood Pressure and Improve Your Overall Health. This book is an essential resource for anybody who wants to take control of their health and hypertension since it contains thorough instructions and advice that is specific to the problem. You will be able to make adjustments to your lifestyle, get an understanding of the many drugs that are available, and take the required actions to lower your blood pressure and enhance the quality of your life with the assistance of this book.

In conclusion, gaining control of hypertension necessitates adopting a multipronged strategy that may include making adjustments to one's lifestyle, taking medicines, engaging in alternative treatments, as well as maintaining frequent monitoring and open communication with one's healthcare practitioner. You may effectively manage your hypertension and enhance your overall health and well-being if you make a commitment to your health and make use of the tools and services that are available to you.

www.ingramcontent.com/pod-product-compliance
Lightning Source LLC
Chambersburg PA
CBHW071145240526
45465CB00024BA/1781